GOODBYE TYPE 2 DIABETES

HOW I REVERSED MY TYPE 2 DIABETES IN 4 MONTHS

A MEMOIR

JOHN D. RODRIGUEZ

FOREWORD

> *Think about it: Heart diseases and diabetes, which account for more deaths in the U.S. and worldwide than everything else combined, are completely preventable by making comprehensive lifestyle changes, without drugs or surgery"-Dean Ornish.*

This quote did not make much sense to me the first time I came across it. "Most diseases like heart disease and diabetes still caught up with people who were living seemingly healthy lives," I thought. I used to belong to the school of thought that believed metabolic diseases were an inevitable part of aging especially if there was already a family history with such medical conditions. So, I didn't bother since I believed that living healthily in early adulthood did not save anyone from diabetes and its cohorts. This orientation guided my way of life for a very long time until reality hit me as I one day, stared at my wife as she slept, for so long that it seemed time stopped. I was so lost in imagining how she would have to go through the rest of the days this world had to offer, alone. Probably, I was more scared that one day, I would breathe my last without a clue of what next would happen to her. I loved this woman so much, and I wanted no harm to come to her, especially if I was going to be the source of the pain. I spent nights wishing that I had not read my obituary even before I crossed death's gates. I had always known I was diabetic and though I was mostly careless about managing my condition, getting to see my condition progress to the point of being referred for various strange tests, dealt me the most significant blow.

I still remember my intestines intertwining the very second Dr. Darbouze told me that my health condition had worsened and that it was likely I would develop pancreatitis if I didn't change my lifestyle. I wondered in that moment why I was so unlucky. I was just beginning to enjoy my life and now I'm being told that I wasn't too far from leaving it permanently. That was in 2009, and I spent several years resigned to the hopelessness of my condition. I bet a lot of people have had similar experiences where they had been told that they had one incurable disease or another which could only be managed.

This is my story. In telling of how I conquered Type 2 diabetes, I felt it was important to relate my background and how I grew up and developed the eating habits that led to having diabetes, and why for many years I resigned myself to this fate. Then, one day was given the hope that I could take control of my life by changing what I was eating. It was though I was drowning and suddenly saw something to grab onto and try to save myself.

1
———

HOME

My name is John Rodriguez, and I was born in Iloilo City, Philippines on March 1967. My parents' marriage did not work out. My father had left my mother and married another woman even before I was born. My mother never remarried and had no other choice, but to raise me and my older sister as a single mother. My Dad visited most times at the close of work before going home to his new family. He kept these visits a secret from his other family. It was during one of such visit that I was conceived. My sister was eighteen years old. And they did continued this relationship intermittently for a few years even after my birth. My dad also helped out financially especially for my sister's college expenses. But the money was always delayed and it wasn't enough and so, my sister was forced to work at the University library so she could get a partial scholarship and have access to free books.

We were poor. My mother and I lived in a small car garage that was converted into a rental place by its owner. It was the cheapest my mother could afford. There was no room in our garage-house but I remember a makeshift partition made of plywood with which we created sections; separating the living room/dining from our room and another barrier that separated the kitchen from the toilet. The exterior of our garage home was made of tin. You could tell that it was due for a paint job because parts of the paint were peeling off. It had two windows made of wood which was rotting from the harsh rays of the sun and rain, and the ceiling was approximately 7 feet high. Due to the nature of the material used in building the garage and the height of the roof which was very low, our house would heat up like an oven during the summer. I didn't even have to move to break a sweat. We did not own an electric fan, and we sure couldn't afford an air conditioner. So we would use an improvised fan made from palm leaves. Those fans were ubiquitous as you would find them in almost every house because they were inexpensive back then and could be readily bought from the market. We had a small black and white television which although was always broken, still served as a decoration of some sort. Amidst all these, our tiny garage was home to us. It was our shelter, and we had already what we needed there. I prided on it as I rarely saw anyone who lived in such a setting. My mother had taught an attitude of always being contented and grateful for the little things I had, into me. And so I was positive about our situation even though I silently wished and prayed that we would have a better and bigger house in the future.

2

GROWING UP

My mother was a typical short Asian woman who was about four feet and eight inches tall. She was not educated enough to find a decent job. Her father had been a poor fisherman while her mother had been a stay-at-home mom who took care of eight children. Her parents could only afford a second-grade education for her, and that made her stop school.

Her lack of proper education barred her from getting any good job so the onus fell on my sister to cater to our needs. Like my grandmother, she was also a stay-at-home mom who did no external jobs because my sister at that time was a working college student who helped mom out, a lot.

After graduation, fortified with her college degree and dreams of escaping the life of poverty, my sister moved to the capital, Manila. She became an employee at a major bank where she would work hard, long hours for bigger paychecks. She has been the sole provider of our little family for as long as I could remember and she made sure I was educated at a private school in town.

Though we were poor, my mother always ensured that what clothes we had were clean. She would wash our clothes by hand for hours. There was no rush whatsoever since she had devoted her time to household chores like washing, cooking and cleaning, while my sister continued to be the bread winner. After the numerous house chores, mom would usually go hangout with her friends Takia and Inga who also lived in our neighborhood. They would smoke cigars from tobacco leaves they hand-rolled as they hung out in the afternoon and gossiped till dawn. This was their daily routine. While I on the other hand, spent the remainder of my day after school, playing hide-and-seek with other kids and sometimes our two dogs.

When I was ten, my sister married her Canadian boyfriend with whom she moved to Montreal, Canada. I noticed she started to send my mother regular monthly allowances which were a little larger than she used to send before her marriage. So we had more money for our rent, food, and my school tuition fees at the private school as well as for miscellaneous expenses. I wasn't sure how much she received from my sister, but my mother was so frugal that we lived like we always didn't have enough money. I didn't have the choice meals the other kids at school used to have. Even the extra snacks they had for the breaks were nothing but items on my wish list. My sister would also send packages which included clothes and goodies every few months. I always looked forward to such packages, it was fun tearing through the packs anticipating new toys, chocolates and stuff.

My family did not own a refrigerator like most of my friends did, so there wasn't enough left-over food all the time. We finished our meals so that it would not spoil since our home was most often than not, very hot. I would say that we were living poorly. My mom liked to cook the dishes that were familiar to her; dishes that she learned from her mother growing up and that always consisted of vegetables and fish. We rarely cooked meat because it was expensive and she only cooked chicken during special occasions like birthdays, Christmas and New Year's Eve.

Lacking the privilege of eating such goodies was dominant in the late seventies till the early eighties and Iloilo City didn't have fast food restaurants. Fast food chains like McDonald's and Dunkin Donuts arrived in the late 80s but then, I didn't have money in my pocket to afford a burger or donuts. We didn't have chips, cookies or fresh milk in the pantry and so, snacking in between meals did not exist for us. Probably these, as well as the fact that I was always outside playing with the neighboring kids until it was dark, were the reasons why I was so skinny. It was easy to read my family's financial situation by merely looking at me. Being fat back then meant that you belonged to a well-off family and the skinny kids were from needy families. Most of my playmates were chubby. They had parents with good jobs and were living well.

3

LAND AWAY FROM HOME: THE MIGRATION

In 1987, when I was 20 and weighed only 115 pounds, my mother and I immigrated to Montreal, Canada to join my sister and her husband. I was so excited when my sister's immigration sponsorship first arrived that I couldn't sleep for a week. I was imagining all the Canadian food I could eat and to finally play in the snow. I was in my first year of nursing and knew I had to drop out of school if I was going to leave, but no second thoughts were given to this as I had been hoping for this for a very long time.

Moving to Montreal was a bit of a culture shock for me. Suddenly, I didn't have any friends, there were no familiar faces and it seemed everyone minded their own business in Montreal. The houses were locked and the whole neighborhood was quiet.

Our new house was also another thing that intrigued me; it was different. It had a refrigerator, microwave and a television that was hooked onto a cable that had so many channels. We even had a basement with a cold cellar and shelves where my sister stocked her groceries and a large freezer which was always filled with frozen meat.

My sister and brother-in-law often had visitors, and for this, we had a supply of assorted wines, cheeses, and European sausages which we kept in the cold cellar in the basement along with the vegetables she harvested from her garden. Our fridge always had a variety of cold cuts for sandwiches and gallons of whole milk which sometimes were kept frozen so that we did not run out of. My sister made sure there was always enough food in the house.

I also noticed something in Canada that I didn't see in the Philippines; there was a barbecue grill on every house's porch. I often wondered if it was a rule because as you looked over people's porches, you were sure to find a barbecue grill. My sister was also fond of barbecuing, so we often had barbecue pork chops, chicken or steak and sometimes lamb chops, on weekends. She taught me how to fire up our gas grill and how to marinate the thick cuts of pork chops with her homemade sauce mixture of mustard, soy sauce, salt, pepper, and lemon. I would brush the sides before turning them over. The marinated meat would sear, and the oil from the fatty layer of the meat would drip on to the hot coal, and its smoke would smell like a medium well steak from Outback Steakhouse. My sister always bought three extra slices because I could eat three or four pieces at a time. I was in heaven! She could well afford to do this as she and her husband both had good paying jobs at the Canadian Marconi Company, a leading electronics company, and so money was never an issue.

This new environment in which I had access to almost any food type I wanted and way of living affected me physically and psychologically. I can't remember how long it took but when I compared my looks at that time to how I looked in previous photos I had made before my mother and I relocated, I was already looking rich as people back in Iloilo City would say. My face was starting to get pudgy. I'm sure it was a result of my daily fresh milk and cheese consumption. I didn't think there was anything wrong about my new seemingly healthy look. I would always run to the toilet thirty minutes later because I was lactose intolerant, although I don't remember having this problem with powdered hot milk back in the Philippines. My mother used to buy powdered milk, which she would dilute in hot water and sweeten it with sugar. I remember closing my eyes when I first drank fresh milk in Montreal; it was so delicious and fresh.

I did not pay attention to my weight. I also did not see a family doctor regularly even though Canadians had a free Medicare. I was in my early twenties and was feeling young and healthy. The mindset of carelessness towards my eating lifestyle was one of the psychological impacts my new environment had on me. Having and eating the kind of meals that I never used to, made me bother less about the possible negative effects they could have on my health.

4

THE ONSET

I did not continue my education for a few reasons: that I lacked English speaking skills, I did not have any friends in school, and I did not consider myself to be a bright student anyway since my grades back in the Philippines was really either failing or very low. I thought I was incapable of doing well in school. I also didn't remember studying my homework since I was more interested in hanging out with my friends and girlfriend. My books were always still new at the end of the school year because I rarely ever touched or opened them to read.

My decision to quit schooling didn't sit well with my sister. She was distraught and suggested that I look for a job and pay rent since I no longer wanted to get a college degree. I could tell that she was very frustrated with my decision because she had always taken care of me since I was born and had worked hard to support my mother and me. She had high hopes for me, but there I was, throwing my future away. It hurt me to see her that way because I loved my sister dearly and admired and respected her for what she had done for our family especially in handling the financial burden. I would have changed my mind and continued with my pursuit for a college degree to make her happy, but I honestly saw all of it as a waste of time because as I had said earlier on, I didn't think I was capable of ever making good grades. So I had to obey my sister's order and apply for jobs that did not require academic qualifications.

In 1988, I found a job at La Gourmand; a French restaurant located a few miles from our place. It was a bit of luck as I had stumbled upon it after combing a couple of blocks one hot afternoon. I found the owners were shorthanded that day because one of the kitchen help had failed to show up. I was put to work immediately, helping in the kitchen and doing the dishes. It was my very first job and so I focused on my tasks to show the owners my value. The owners practically begged me to come back the next day, and that was how I started working for them. A couple of days later, my brother-in-law bought me a bicycle with which I would bike to work every day except on snowy days. On such days, I took the bus to work. I worked in the kitchen with Gilles, a chef that had just moved to Montreal from France, where I learned more about French-Canadian cuisine. My favorite was the Reuben Sandwich. It had a pound of smoked-meat, sauerkraut sautéed in garlic butter and a slice of Swiss cheese. Another favorite of mine was the Pioneer sandwich; a foot-long French bread with some garlic butter spread, a generous amount of Canadian bacon over it, oven-baked Swiss cheese and a few slices of tomatoes added to it before being eaten. I was allowed to eat anytime in the kitchen and so, I did. The young owners were very generous to the entire staff. I reckon that I must have gained a few more pounds while working there as well but I still did not go to the doctor for a checkup because my weight didn't bother me at all. It was a beautiful transition and a new identity seeing as skinny wasn't appreciated back home in the Philippines. More so, my new love or obsession as I would instead call it, for food was enough to keep my mind from worrying about how bad an overweight body could be for my health.

In 1989, I eventually made some friends and decided to move out of my sister's place and into a two-bedroom apartment which I rented with a friend. This way, I could come home anytime I wanted no matter how late it was. I had always loved to party at the local bars with friends, but I couldn't satisfy this craving while still under my sister's roof. I also didn't have to do household chores, and this new found freedom made that possible. When I lived with my sister, she made me do tasks, and I hated it but did not complain because she was older and I was brought up not to talk back to my elders. The only chore I didn't have to do was cook the food because my sister prepared our meals all the time. When I moved out to live on my own, I didn't cook most of the time since I was alone and my apartment was near Harvey's burger joint, so I would always eat fast food. I also bought a barbecue grill for the weekends when my friends would visit. They usually had a case of twenty-four beers with them.

Later on, I quit working at the restaurant to work at Electropac Canada, an electronics factory making printed circuit boards. The factory was two blocks away from my apartment, and it operated a shifting regime. My shift schedule in my first month at Electropac was the second shift that began at three-thirty p.m. and ended at eleven p.m. I would arrive home thirty minutes later and hungry. The restaurants were usually closed at those hours, so I would cook a can of corned beef that I kept in the pantry, with lots of garlic and onions. I would eat the above with 3-4 cups of steamed white rice all by myself. If I got bored with corned beef, I would fry a pack of a dozen hotdogs or a can of spam. I would finish my dinner by two o'clock a.m., after which I would watch the television until I fell asleep, most often, around four o'clock am. I had gradually developed a cycle: habitually eating, staying up, and sleeping late. I was putting myself at higher risk of weight gain and Type 2 diabetes, and I didn't even know it. This pattern continued for two years until my work shift schedule was changed to the morning shift. I had already gained a lot of weight at that time and even worse was that I moved closer to my workplace. This proximity between my house and my workplace meant that I would no longer exercise as much as I did when compared to when I biked a few miles to the restaurant at which I formerly worked. Still, there was no seeing a doctor, no exercise, a lot of partying, excessive amounts of alcohol, more late night meals and more sleeping-in late. Having my freedom allowed me to do whatever

I wanted. I occasionally smoked pot with friends, and even though I silently wished for some little restraint, there was no one to stop me. Sometimes, I tried to create mental scenarios of how my mother and sister would react if they somehow found me living that way. I would always shrug off imaginations of my brother-in-law admonishing me disapprovingly, on how such irresponsible living could never come in handy in raising and managing a family of my own. Deep down within, I was not proud of the path I had found myself on, but it was fun at the time, and fun was what mattered to a single man. After a childhood filled with abject poverty, I was determined to get all the fun I could of life, I was determined to enjoy it to the fullest. This was supposed to be the life, after all.

5
____

HEAVEN'S BLESSING

I still believe a God somewhere, or maybe a guardian angel saw through me and how I quietly wished I were living healthier. I say this because, in 1999, I met Armie on one of my vacations to the Philippines. She lived there and had the cutest smile and most beautiful skin like I had never seen. Her face was not at all puffy, but one could see that she was healthy and full of life. Her family was wealthy but she was slender. She was very conscious about making healthy food choices. Armie and I would spend hours talking about everything and nothing.

Everything ranged from what she would consider as the peak of her career and her plans to get there, to the number of kids she would like to have and if she wouldn't mind moving away from the Philippines and for what reason it would be. The nothings were the times we would be in each other's company with no words in between, just the assurance that we shared a bond which we had come to see as designed by fate and all the forces on the earth and beyond. Armie was a physician specializing in Internal Medicine and just recently started her private practice when I came into her life.

Our love grew so much that we couldn't imagine living apart and so we got married in the Philippines, a year after we first met. She was willing to relocate to Montreal with me, and so we left to build our small unit of the universe which we vowed to cherish. She was a vegetarian but started eating more meat when we began living together since I preferred to eat meat especially pork. Eventually, I stopped hanging out with my friends and gradually changed my eating and sleeping habits to healthier routines. I even quit smoking, and I can bet that Armie was mainly responsible for this new way of life. Although she would have loved a onetime end to my alcohol consumption, I still enjoyed drinking and barbecue on weekends at home. She would always remind me of the dangers of alcohol to my liver, but I ignored it.

6

SOFT WARNING SIGNALS

In 2003, I quit working at the factory and went back to school because I realized that I was becoming more interested in computers and website design. So, I enrolled at the International Academy of Design and Technology in Montreal to get a degree in Digital Multimedia Design. I badly wanted to become a website designer especially as I had taken enough of the factory job; I was receiving a meager salary that was getting me nowhere, and most importantly, I didn't want Armie to think that I was a loser for dropping out of college. She never did say this though, but a part of me was sure that it had crossed her mind at least, twice. I was bothered about this and wanted her to be proud of me. She also wanted to continue her career as a physician in Montreal, but we later discovered that it was impossible for International Medical Graduates to become doctors in Quebec. And so, my wife and I moved to Jersey City, New Jersey in 2006 for better opportunities since Montreal had nothing for her. Quebec is a French-speaking province, and it was impossible for us to get decent jobs since we lacked French-speaking proficiency.

With my website design skills on my shoulder, I was able to find a job in New York City. My wife had a Bachelor's degree in Nursing, so she got a job as well at the hospital, and we were both working. My wife and I temporarily stayed with her brother Arsenio in West Side Avenue, Jersey City. Arsenio was renting a two-bedroom apartment located on the street where many Filipinos lived. That neighborhood made one feel like they were walking on the streets of Manila. I could smell the same air as I would in the Philippines. Maybe this was possible as there was a Filipino restaurant in every corner and they all had the aroma of native Filipino dishes wafting through their kitchens. The one across our apartment was named Apollo restaurant. We ate there almost every day because it was more convenient and cheaper; six dollars a plate and that got you two cups of rice, two types of dishes and a free soda. And the plethora of Filipino dishes in their selection was plenty, mostly meat choices especially pork swimming in oily sauce and so greasy that even the Filipinos invented a joke that went by our local language, "Pampabata," meaning "to live young." It was a regular joke in our culture which meant that the food you were eating was so bad for your heart that you could not reach old age because you would surely die young from a heart attack. I have seen and heard Filipinos that were regular customers suffering from heart attacks and dialysis but I didn't think at the time that diet was the root cause of their diseases. Filipino food has a strong Spanish influence because Spain colonized the Republic of the Philippines for three hundred and thirty-three years. This reflected in Filipino culture and especially in the names of most of our foods such as lechon, a slow-roasted suckling pig; adobo, meat marinated in a sauce made of vinegar, soy sauce, and spices; chicharron, a delicious piece of fried pork skin crackling; empanadas, meat-filled pastries shaped like a half circle, embutido, and many others.

Dr. Caldwell Esselstyn, heart surgeon and author of *"Prevent and Reverse Heart Disease,"* asserts that eating meat, eggs, dairy, fish and oily foods, injures the capacity of the endothelium to make nitric oxide. Nitric oxide is very important because it expands the blood vessels, increasing blood flow to the heart and decreasing plaque growth and blood clotting. When the endothelium senses high cholesterol, high blood pressure, or smoking, it releases less nitric oxide, and atherosclerosis (heart disease) accelerates. Dr. Esselstyn also said that, "the types of bacteria in our gut depends on what we eat. Meat eaters have bacteria in their gut that metabolizes the meat products into Trimethylamine (TMA). The TMA will be rapidly oxidized by your liver into Trimethylamine N–oxide (TMAO). TMAO raises havoc with your blood vessels causing vascular disease."

West Side Avenue also had many African-Americans and Latinos living in the neighborhood and located within too were the McDonald's, Dunkin Donuts and Popeye's fried-chicken takeout joints. It was very common to see an obese or overweight person every day. And I think it contributed to one of the many reasons why my excessive weight seemed reasonable to me. I felt it was entirely rational and even better since I fitted well into the environment, unlike when I was skinny in Iloilo City where I stood out so distinctly. Another reason was that these unhealthy foods were also cheap and worked perfectly for the budget my wife and I was on.

As a website designer, I spent numerous hours sitting in front of my computer, working on a project and I consumed unlimited amounts of coffee, soda, fruit juices and chips as I worked. I also did not exercise because I had neither the desire nor the energy to do so. I would later go on to find out in one of my research that the Mayo Clinic asserts that research had linked sitting for long periods of time with a number of health concerns, including obesity and metabolic syndrome, a cluster of conditions that included increased blood pressure, high blood sugar, excess body fat around the waist and abnormal cholesterol levels. Too much sitting also seemed to increase the risk of death from cardiovascular disease, but I was not aware of this back then. I knew that becoming a website designer entailed many hours of coding in front of my computer and I loved my work. I also noticed my lack of energy when taking the stairs or while suddenly running to seek shelter from the rain. I would feel faint and out of breath every time I made a sudden movement that required any form of energy. My knees hurt painfully whenever I bent or sat down to pick something up. I noticed these signs and other little warnings my body gave. I preferred to bury my head in the sand. I believed that if I didn't bother with these pesky disturbances, they would go away on their own. My body was flashing a red light warning but I ignored the signs, because I thought these things came with aging. At this time, I was already in my forties.

THE DISCOVERY

In 2007, I could no longer ignore my failing health, it simply wasn't going away. So I went to the hospital for a check up and I was diagnosed with Type 2 Diabetes. My Hemoglobin A1c (HbA1c) was 12.5%, and by the standard range levels, I was confirmed to be a diabetic. The hemoglobin A1c test could evaluate your average level of blood sugar over the past 2 to 3 months and could be employed in determining if you had diabetes or not. People who were not diabetic had the normal range for the hemoglobin A1c level which is between 4% and 5.6%. Hemoglobin A1c levels between 5.7% and 6.4% meant that you were pre-diabetic. Concentrations of 6.5% or higher meant that you had diabetes.

My wife's face turned pale with concern. I could not tell what exactly was on her mind, but I saw her fears assume form and life. I remember becoming very worried because I had relatives and friends who lost their eyesight and limbs to Diabetes Mellitus. The thought of this happening to me later in life bothered me somewhat, however, it seemed like I was in a bubble wrap because the reality didn't sink in.

Dr. Jean Darbouze, my new family doctor, was a Haitian-American who spoke with a French accent. He had a well-built body structure, and you would almost believe he had no troubles or life challenges as he had a confident and calm demeanor. He was friendly, always smiling and he laughed a lot. His great personality helped put me at ease somewhat. He prescribed Metformin, a blood sugar control pill, and Lipitor, to regulate my cholesterol level after counseling me on how I needed to develop new habits like eating healthy and then encouraged me to meticulously observe my new drug routine. I could tell he sensed my spirit was washed and went on to say to me that I could live longer with proper management of the condition. Unlike in Canada, healthcare was not free in America, but I was lucky that my wife was working in the hospital as a registered nurse, so she had a good insurance plan which had me included in it.

Having Type 2 Diabetes felt normal; there were no apparent symptoms, no hurting or anything out of the ordinary. Apart from the usual symptoms (which appeared normal for a man my age), I felt fine. Armie pointed out other signs such as going to the bathroom at night to urinate, but that had appeared normal until I was diagnosed with diabetes. I think in fact, that many people with Type 2 Diabetes or pre-diabetes do not even know that they have it and this is primarily because they would only go for a medical checkup when they felt sick.

I was also having frequent dreams and a lot of sleep talking. I would also often sleepwalk to the bathroom and wouldn't remember why I went to the bathroom when I got there. Armie was supportive and understanding even though I contributed to her sleepless nights with my new night activities. She informed me that diabetes could affect my eyes, heart, kidneys, brain and blood vessels if I did not control my drinking and eating habits. I did not heed her caution however and continued to eat what I considered regular food then, which some doctors called the Standard American Diet (SAD). It might also interest you to know that a typical Filipino breakfast would be some hotdogs, corned beef, and eggs over fried rice or steamed white rice. I also enjoyed drinking alcohol almost every Friday evening with my co-workers because I had always been a social person. As the days turned into months and the months turned into years, I began to forget that I was ill. I was back to my old habits of eating at fast food restaurants, having more Chinese buffets than I needed, barbecue on weekends and drinking excessive amounts of alcohol. Armie would always be upset every time I came home drunk because she was worried for my health knowing that I had diabetes. She would always remind me of how diabetes was capable of affecting my blood vessels and nerves and how I could have my system shut down if I continued neglecting my health. She kept nagging me about this every time I had a drink after work, and this was usually every Friday. I don't know why I never listened to her, early enough. Probably, I had prioritized having fun partying in New York City with my British co-workers at Ulysses bar on Wall Street, over my slowly failing health.

In 2008, my wife and I bought our condominium. Armie had always wanted one especially as she wanted more space and privacy. Our new acquisition was on a quiet street about three miles away from West Side Avenue. There were no restaurants nearby, but I later found out that our new neighborhood also had a large concentration of Filipinos and I was glad to discover that my next-door neighbor was a Filipino who also worked at a liquor store. His name was Chris, and he and I became friends almost instantly. Occasionally, we would have drinks with his friends in our back garage which was adjacent. Chris was so skilled in cooking barbecue; I felt he should have opened a barbecue joint, but he was only interested in sharing his culinary skills with his family and friends. He always offered me whatever he was grilling — pork, sausage, beef or fish. We would have a couple of cases of beer and a big bottle of vodka that he brought from his workplace. Chris liked to drink vodka shots with beer all night, and I was right there with him drinking and eating. Deep inside I knew this was not good for my health condition but Chris and his friends were great guys who were fun to be with, so I continued ignoring the health risks in exchange for the fun. Besides, I didn't have to worry about driving home since I lived next door.

8

WALKING INTO THE LION'S LAIR

In 2009, Dr. Darbouze ordered another blood work, and the results showed that my HbA1c was 7.4 and my triglyceride was 174. The ideal range for triglyceride is 0-149. My triglyceride levels were way higher than the typical range. Dr. Darbouze became increasingly concerned for my health this time. He knew I hadn't been taking care of my health and told me that if I continued drinking alcohol that I could end up with pancreatitis. It didn't ring a bell to me because I didn't know what pancreatitis was. I looked at Armie, and she was almost in tears.

On the drive home from the doctor's, Armie explained to me that pancreatitis is the inflammation of the pancreas and that it could cause pancreatic cancer or kidney failure. She explained what patients with kidney failures went through during dialysis and it did not sound pleasant to me, at all. I admitted that I was scared and promised Armie and myself that I was going to stop consuming alcohol. I continued with this resolution for a couple of months until that day when Chris was cooking barbecue from his garage again. I perceived the smell of smoke wafting from the drops of the barbecue sauce on the hot coals of the grill and onto my nostrils, every time the wind blew in my direction where I was standing. I opened my garage door to confirm the source of this enticing smell. Just about the same time I stuck my neck out, Chris greeted me with a smile. His friends, Nilo and Lambert had visited and been watching as Chris fanned the half-done pork chops and steaks while holding a cold beer in their hands. I greeted the guys. I had missed their company, the funny stories, the delicious cooked barbecue pork and steak dipped in garlic vinegar, the cold Coors Light beer and the intermittent rounds of vodka shots. The guys invited me to unwind, and so I went closer. I noticed the red cooler sitting just beside the garage door, looked inside and saw that there were plenty of beers. Suddenly, I became thirsty. It was a Friday afternoon, and our Friday drinking sessions were repeated every so often since then.

My negligence towards my health was causing more havoc than the actual disease itself. I still had Type 2 Diabetes, and my condition was not improving. So I was just going through life with Type 2 Diabetes and medications, which now included insulin injections to my stomach, twice daily. However, I still felt normal as though I was without diabetes; there were still no symptoms. I remember thinking I could afford to eat whatever I wanted since I was on medication. I reasoned the drugs were going to keep my blood sugar levels from shooting up into the sky. I was eating cakes, soda, chocolate bars, big pieces of cheeses, snacks at Popeye's chicken, Big Macs at McDonald's, large slices of pizza. I didn't check my blood glucose levels because I was afraid of what it would read since I had been eating meals that had high sugar content. I am sure some diabetic patients still have this type of attitude towards their eating habits. Going on to eat just anything as a diabetic patient was one of the most harmful and dangerous things a person could do for their health. While the medication may make one think everything was under control, everything wasn't.

&

9

DIM LIGHTS FLOODING IN

In 2015, I decided to change careers because I didn't love website design anymore. I'd had to change employers every year, and each time my salary was back where it started. I realized then that there was an endless supply of web design professionals in New York and employers were fond of choosing the ones that had the most and current skills and that were willing to work for less money. I hated having to work more extended hours to complete projects without any compensation or increase in my pay. Worse still, every employer I had worked for offered no medical insurance. So I decided to pursue my nursing degree that I had paused for many years. My primary motivation for this move was my wife's take-home pay that was three times more than what I made as a web designer. I thought having a nurse's salary would help make our lives even more comfortable if both of us were earning decent money.

So I enrolled at Hudson County Community College in Jersey City. I was forty-eight years old already, and most of my classmates were decades younger than me; the rest were just a few students who were my age-mates. Science was not my favorite course back when I was in school but there I was again with it, staring me in the face. Once again I learned about the cells, hormones, blood, organs, and everything about the human body in our Anatomy & Physiology course, as well as in our Microbiology classes. I learned that every time we eat, food especially carbohydrates gets converted into glucose which is then released into the blood. Then, our pancreas releases a hormone called insulin, which creates a passage that allows the glucose to enter the cells for energy production. We were also taught that glucose is one of the leading energy sources for our body and that if insulin was not produced or appropriately released, glucose will remain and persist in our bloodstream and that was how Type 2 Diabetes could develop. We also learned about the different systems such as the cardiovascular system, nervous system, circulatory system, and lymphatic system. I was interested in these topics because I did understand them better as an adult compared to when I was a teenager. I also had Type 2 Diabetes, and so I was paying complete attention to the lectures as well as having personal study sessions. In one of my study periods, I learned that diabetes is a group of metabolic diseases characterized by the presence of high concentration of glucose or sugar in the blood as a result of problems with insulin production or secretion. This insulin is said to be a hormone released by the pancreas, a gland near the stomach, and it is responsible for facilitating the usage and storage of sugar and fat have gotten from the food we eat, by the cells of the body. I read that whenever the pancreas can no longer produce insulin or produces very little or whenever the body does not respond appropriately to the insulin (a condition referred to as insulin resistance), diabetes and its complications were said to be at play as insulin is crucial for regulating blood sugar levels. Various articles I came across agreed that there are several types of diabetes which included Type 1 Diabetes in which there is no insulin production by the pancreas, and it could be developed in teenage years or early adulthood. Type 2 Diabetes is characterized by the little production of insulin, which is insufficient for the proper functioning of the cells, or insulin resistance in which the body does not respond to the insulin produced. This type of diabetes is said to be progressive; meaning that the patient will eventually need to depend on insulin injections for the rest of their lives.

Lifestyle choices, especially diet and weight gain are a crucial factor in Type 2 Diabetes, which often sets in with advancement in a person's age (typically 40 years old). Other risks of developing this form of diabetes increases with, obesity, and lack of physical activity. Gestational diabetes is another type of diabetes, which usually arises, in pregnant women who probably had meals high in animal fat and cholesterol. Symptoms of diabetes differ from one diabetes type to another. For Type 1 Diabetes, symptoms ranged from increased thirst and hunger (especially after eating), dry mouth, frequent urination to loss of consciousness (which is usually rare). For Type 2 Diabetes, there are no symptoms; however, there is a very gradual development of Type 1 Diabetes symptoms as well as slow-healing sores or cuts, and weight gain. I also read that diabetes is a lifelong disease that had no cure. I didn't like this new information because it had me wondering if taking medications weren't a waste of time and resources since there was no cure for my condition. I was beginning to accept that I was never going to live a medication-free life, but then, I loved life and living would entail having to take pills, so I chose to live, rather than taking pills. If I had been told that diabetes could be cured, I would have staked bets on it that it was impossible because it was tough to find any article that didn't mention that diabetes is incurable.

10

WAVING THE WHITE FLAG

In November 2016, I was back at Dr. Darbouze's office for more blood work. After the tests, my Hemoglobin A1c was 9.9% which were still very high. In fact, it had increased compared to the test result I had at the previous blood work.

Dr. Darbouze observed that my heart was beating faster than usual and was trying to think of the possible reasons why my heart was beating fast when he asked if I was taking drugs or smoking cigarettes. I replied no to both questions, but I lied about smoking cigarettes. My wife was in the room, and it would break her heart to find out that I had been smoking cigarettes, occasionally. I felt guilty for lying, mainly because my health was never getting better and she was worried sick about it. The doctor wrote down Metoprolol, a beta-blocker which makes the heart beat slower and decreases the blood pressure. My medications went from two to six drug types. The insulin injections continued, and I did not like the needles to my stomach; it was never easy, and it terrified me every time because it hurt badly, leaving bruises at the injection site after a while. I was beginning to worry because I had been taking these medications for ten years and yet, I was still sick. At this point, I had completely accepted that I would have to be on medication for the rest of my life.

I didn't even question my doctor about when I could stop taking the medicines because people said that Type 2 Diabetes is a disease that progressed with age and I had read that once a person had it, that person had it for life. I just trusted Dr. Darbouze because he had been managing my condition since I walked into his office in 2007, but then, doctors couldn't help so much if a patient wasn't helping themselves. It was entirely up to that patient to take control of their health. As for diabetes, a doctor could only guide on how to control or manage blood glucose level with medication, but it was the patient who had the task of identifying the source of why or how they got sick in the first place and avoiding such things that they found to be responsible for it, if they were avoidable.

11

———

THE SCARE

In December of 2016, Dr. Darbouze's office was moved to a new location in Jersey City. It was impossible to find parking at the new place, so I decided to see a different doctor with parking and closer to where I lived. Dr. Dilruba Khanam's office was a few blocks away from my house. She refilled my prescriptions and suggested that I needed to do a colonoscopy especially as I had advanced in age. Having to go through such test procedures terrified me much because I heard that colonoscopy involved the insertion of a tube into the anus to examine if the colon was in good health. I was determined not to have this procedure because I didn't want any foreign object to penetrate my anus. The thought of it terrified me. So I told the doctor that I would think about it. The new doctor gave me three months' worth of medications including referrals to a podiatrist who was to check the nerves on my lower limbs and another reference to an ophthalmologist for the examination of my eyes. These, the doctor said, were to investigate if I had developed diabetic complications. Such knowledge was going to help manage whatever the difficulties were, early enough so I wouldn't have to lose vital organs.

I was concerned about these referrals because I didn't want bad news. Bad news at that time would have read: Dear Mr. John, we may have to have your legs amputated to avoid further damage to other parts of your limbs. Your left eye is incapable of functioning any longer, and we may have to conduct surgery to manage your right eye before it deteriorates. At least, that was how I imagined the report in my head. So I decided to leave my head buried in the sand.

The skin on my legs was already turning darker like they had been sunburnt and my eyesight was getting worse; I experienced great pains in my eyes which made them tear each time I read for anytime longer than 30 minutes. At this point, I knew that my Type 2 Diabetes was progressing rapidly and that I had to do something about it but I had no idea what steps to take. I continued with my medications, however, and this time, I became more serious about the routines because it had dawned on me that I could be very close to the end stage of this disease.

12

THE BREAKTHROUGH

June 24, 2017 is a day I will never forget. It was the day light shone through the dark tunnel of my state of helplessness, and it marked the beginning of my health condition's turn-around. On this day I decided to completely change my lifestyle after watching a Netflix documentary titled, "What the Health." The movie opened my mind to the adverse health impact of meat and dairy products consumption to our body. It was the best eye-opening documentary I had ever watched.

"What the Health" was a documentary by filmmaker, Kip Andersen and it uncovered the secret to preventing and even reversing chronic diseases. In the documentary, Andersen investigated why the nation's leading health organizations don't reveal this knowledge to the public. The movie started with Hippocrates' quote, "Let food be thy medicine and medicine be thy food," which was immediately followed by a scene that had Andersen interviewing Robert Ratner, Chief Scientific & Medical Officer of the American Diabetes Association.

In that interview, Dr. Ratner said that we are in the midst of a diabetes epidemic and there are approximately three hundred and fifteen million people living with diabetes worldwide. He also said that one in three Medicare dollars was spent in the care of people with diabetes and that one in ten total health care dollar was spent on people with diabetes.

"There's no question that this is a major problem," he said.

Andersen then asked Dr. Ratner a follow-up question about the correlation between diets and diabetes and to my surprise, Dr. Ratner replied, "I'm not going to get into that."

I couldn't believe what I had just watched. I didn't expect such answer from the Chief Scientific & Medical Officer of the American Diabetes Association. As a type 2 diabetic myself, I felt that they knew something that we didn't know of and that Andersen knew and was trying to expose or reveal this information to the public. This spiked my curiosity and I continued watching with keen interest. The documentary proceeded with Kip Anderson relating information about his background; about how he was a recovering hypochondriac and how his family had a history of diabetes, heart diseases, and cancer. He had lost his grandfather to diabetes, and both other grandparents to cancer and so had been trying to live a healthy lifestyle all his life by exercising regularly, not smoking, avoiding soda, taking vitamin supplements. In short, he had been all about taking good care of himself to avoid getting sick. Well, that was until he saw an episode on the Today's News that showed that the World Health Organization had classified red meat as group 2 carcinogens and processed meat such as bacon and sausage as carcinogenic and that it could be as dangerous as smoking cigarettes; and directly involved in causing cancer in humans. His research also found out that the World Health Organization had analyzed 800 studies from ten different countries and experts had concluded that each 50-gram portion of processed meat eaten daily increased the risk of colorectal cancer by 18%. And then he suddenly realized that processed meat included hotdogs, bacon, sausage, salami, ham, pepperoni, cold cuts and deli slices, basically everything we grew up eating. Andersen said that the World Health Organization classified processed meat as a Group One carcinogen; the same group as cigarettes, asbestos, and plutonium. And then he thought about his kids, "If processed meats have been labeled the same as cigarettes, how was it even legal for kids to be eating such foods?" he asked.

13

AND THE SCALES FELL OFF

fter finding out how dangerous processed meat is to our body, Andersen went to the American Cancer Society's website and was shocked to see that none of these information was on their website and even more shocking for him was the fact that their "Eat Healthy" page was encouraging the public to eat processed meat such as canned tuna, salmon, minced clams and chicken; the same foods that the World Health Organization labeled as Group One carcinogens. I immediately put the documentary on pause and made some coffee. This information was new to me and I wanted to know every bit of it. I resumed the movie after I had my cup of coffee ready. Andersen was now trying to setup an interview with someone from the American Cancer Society and he was scheduled to go but his interview got cancelled when he told them that his interview was about the correlation between diet and cancer.

Wait now, I said to myself, I'm really seeing a pattern here— diet; food; processed meat and cancer, I finished. I took a sip of my coffee and continued to watch.

When the American Cancer Society representative kept avoiding Andersen without any explanation for the indefinite postponement, he searched for answers elsewhere and found a group of doctors who were willing to talk about the link between our food and metabolic diseases.

The first doctor he interviewed was Dr. Alan Goldhamer, the founder of True North Health Center in Santa Rosa, California; a state-of-the-art facility that provides medical and chiropractic services, psychotherapy and counseling. He was also said to be the Director of the Center's groundbreaking residential health education program. Dr. Goldhamer asserted that we were creating an epidemic cascade of debilitating diseases with our diet and lifestyle choices and he also talked about how two-thirds of adults were either overweight or obese.

The second doctor Andersen interviewed was Dr. Joel Kahn, a summa cum laude graduate of the University Of Michigan School Of Medicine. His profile read that he practices cardiology in Detroit and is a clinical professor of medicine at Wayne State University School of Medicine. Dr. Kahn also asserted that diabetes; arthritis, heart diseases, dementia, obesity, and cancers were responsible for about 70% of deaths and all the data showed that they were largely lifestyle related and preventable.

Dr. Michael Greger was also interviewed. Dr. Greger is a physician, bestselling author, leading nutrition expert, and an internationally recognized speaker on a number of important public health issues. He is a founding member and Fellow of the American College of Lifestyle Medicine and founder of nutritionfacts.org; a website dedicated to providing nutritional information. Dr. Greger claimed that most ten-year-old kids in America already had fatty streaks in their arteries; this marks the first stage of atherosclerosis leading to heart attacks and strokes.

The next interviewee was Dr. Milton Mill, a Stanford University School of Medicine graduate, an internist and a Critical Care Physician in Inova Fairfax Hospital. Major focuses of Dr. Mills' patient advisement as well as his lecturing involve the use of nutritional measures to reduce the risk of major chronic diseases. Dr. Mills maintained that American medicine operate from the disease model. "Medicine is in the business of treating sick people and they are not in the business of preventing people from becoming sick." he said.

Dr. Michelle McMacken, an honors graduate of Yale University and Columbia University College of Physicians and Surgeons, was also interviewed. She has had more than ten years of experience practicing primary care, and teaching doctors-in-training at Bellevue Hospital Center in New York. A board-certified internal medicine physician and an assistant professor of medicine at NYU School of Medicine, she said, "Dietary choices trumps smoking when it comes to chronic disease risk."

Anderson also interviewed Dr. Michael Klaper, a graduate of the University Of Illinois College Of Medicine in Chicago who has more than 40 years experience having served as an advisor to the National Aeronautics and Space Administration (NASA) project on nutrition for long-term space colonists on the moon and Mars. Dr. Klaper confirmed that the cause of diabetes and clogged arteries, high blood pressure and obesity is the food. "It's what the Americans are eating," he said while referring to the Standard American Diet.

Andersen continued, saying that one in three Americans would have diabetes in the next twenty-five years and that the government and media would not stop blaming the lack of exercise and sugary foods as the cause. So he went on to interview a diabetes expert and researcher, Dr. Neal Barnard.

Dr. Barnard is President of the Physicians Committee for Responsible Medicine; a fellow of the American College of Cardiology, the 2016 recipient of the American College of Lifestyle Medicine's Trailblazer Award, and has led numerous research studies investigating the effects of diet on diabetes, body weight, and chronic pain, including a groundbreaking study of dietary interventions in Type 2 Diabetes, funded by the National Institutes of Health. The best explanation and most detailed explanation that I understood and what stuck with me was Dr. Neal Barnard's response to Anderson's question on what role sugar played in causing diabetes.

Here is that response: "Diabetes is not and never was caused by eating a high carbohydrate diet and sugar. The cause of diabetes is a diet; a meat-based or animal-based diet to be exact, that builds up a high amount of fat into the blood. It is the buildup of tiny particles of fat into the muscle cells of the human body that's causing insulin resistance. This buildup of fat in our cells is called Intramyocellular lipid. This means that the sugar that's naturally from the food that we're eating can't get into our cells where it belongs. It builds up in our blood and that's diabetes."

14

THE TURNING POINT

I had grown up thinking that eating too much sugary food and drinks caused diabetes because I heard random people repeat this claim over and over, although these people were not doctors. I had also always believed that diabetes could never be cured. This documentary was however, revealing something new and interestingly, it was coming from an expert American diabetes doctor. I believed Dr. Barnard and I was determined to apply what I had heard him say and to see its effects on my diabetic condition.

A few more doctors were also interviewed; I wrote down their names so I could do more research about them on my own. Hearing these many doctors single-mindedly affirm the link between meat consumption and its negative impact on our health, cemented my belief that I had to self-experiment and stop eating all meat products for a month, just to see what happens. I had been absorbing this new information and taking notes that would serve to guide the experiments I planned to conduct on and by myself. I also realized that our typical Filipino breakfast, which was always consisted of either hotdog or spam with fried rice, was rich in processed meat, which I never imagined was carcinogenic until I came across the documentary. I cancelled that out of our meal plan. Andersen showed a research finding from Harvard that one serving of processed meat per day increased the risk of developing diabetes by 51 percent. It became glaring that my diabetic condition had some roots in my love for meat and its products. I started solving puzzles in my mind; calculating how all the meat I had consumed especially after I moved to Montreal, must have led to my diabetic condition.

In the movie, Andersen went to the American Diabetes Association website and showed that they were featuring recipes for red and processed meat. I could not take this because it sounded blasphemous. "How could it be possible that a body tasked with helping people manage their diabetic condition would encourage the very practices that were the frontline cause for the disease itself?" I asked. So I pressed pause on my remote and straightaway, visited www.diabetes.org. I clicked on Food & Fitness, Recipes, and did a search on "Pork" in their recipes page and I was surprised to see Smoky Pork Chops with Tomatoes - Recipes for Healthy Living by the American Diabetes Association.

I was dazed and completely lost in thoughts, wondering who was right between Dr. Neal Barnard and the American Diabetes Association. I got curious and clicked on the "About Us" page and there sat a bold "We lead the fight against the deadly consequences of diabetes and fight for those affected by diabetes. We fund research to prevent, cure and manage diabetes. We deliver services to hundreds of communities. We provide objective and credible information. We give voice to those denied their rights because of diabetes." This, I thought, was far from the damaging implications of the information people were accessing from their website.

Now I really had to find out who was telling the truth. I decided that self-experimentation using this new knowledge from these doctors especially Dr. Barnard's, was going to be the tool for knowing who was right or wrong. The documentary had left a big impact on me and so, I started with researching on these doctors. I searched online and also found plenty YouTube video presentations of them and was obsessed for weeks, watching most of their videos talk about the positive health impact of whole food plant-based diets on humans. I came across more doctors who inspired me such as Dr. John McDougall, Dr. Caldwell Esselstyn, and Dr. T. Collin Campbell who wrote a book entitled, "The China Study."

I followed these doctors on YouTube and played their video in my kitchen every time I prepared my dog's meal and ours as well.

I decided to stop eating all meat products including fish and I resolved that I was going to do it cold turkey. I knew it was going to be difficult but I had spent so much on medications that I was not even religiously taking. There had been no improvement and at least, avoiding meat seemed a better choice than having painful needles to my stomach, two times every day. Armie was very supportive. The change was not going to be drastic for her, I would say, since she had been a vegetarian at the time before we got married and moved to Montreal. She was even excited because her clothes were starting to feel tighter. She didn't like it that she had started to put on more weight.

I went and opened our refrigerator's freezer compartment and saw quite a few frozen chicken parts, pork, processed meat and a pint of chocolate ice cream. I emptied them all out, transferred them to a box and gave them to my brother-in-law. He was not vegan and I hated to throw food away. It would be like throwing money away and that was not a leisure we could afford; my medical bills were already piling up by the side. I checked the rest of the fridge and pantry and everything with dairy in it went straight to the garbage. My favorite strong cheddars, dry cured sausages, mayonnaise, bread with egg in its ingredient, eggs, salad dressings and a gallon of milk also went into the garbage. It was the most liberating feeling and it reminded me of what I felt when I decided to quit smoking and had to give away a pack of cigarettes. It was that feeling of taking back full control of your life as well as all the choices.

15

THE BIG QUESTION

Then, the big question came. What was I going to be eating? All my life, I had been cooking food recipes that had strong meat influence. Suddenly, all I had were vegetables and more vegetables. I remembered I had browsed for some plant-based recipes a week before and smoothies were the easier option at that time. I was curious about a particular smoothie recipe called TropiKale and I had a reason to try it since I was clueless on what to do with the vegetables I was left with. TropiKale is a blend of raw kale leaves, baby spinach, pineapple slices, banana and almond milk. I drove to the supermarket and chose the organic kale and baby spinach since I would be eating them raw. I had also read about farmers using heavy pesticides on their crops and although I couldn't prove that organic crops weren't being sprayed with pesticides, it made me feel better that they were at least organic and that I was not deliberately ingesting poison (in my opinion). I used the regular non-organic bananas and pineapples because I didn't find any organic ones at that time. And besides, I could peel off the outer layer of the fruit anyway. My first TropiKale smoothie was a success. It was delicious and Armie loved it as well. We talked about how it tasted and felt on our taste buds that we decided to make it an everyday meal in our kitchen and it had been that way, ever since. I also convinced Armie to invest in a professional blender to which I dropped $500 on a new Blendtec blender I found on eBay. Since the blender arrived, I have made over five hundred smoothies to date because kale and spinach had to be consumed in our home, every day. I searched online and went to WebMD's website for the benefits of kale and I found out that one cup of raw kale has only 33 calories, approximately 3 grams of protein, vitamins A, C, and K, 2.5 grams of fiber (which helps manage blood sugar and makes you feel full), folate, a B vitamin that's key for brain development, alpha-linolenic acid, omega-3 fatty acid, lutein and zeaxanthin which protects against macular degeneration and cataracts, and finally, minerals like phosphorus, potassium, calcium, and zinc.

My joy was boundless when I read that kale was very effective in improving the health of the human eyes. The National Institute of Health had described diabetic eye disease as a group of eye conditions that could affect people with diabetes. A number of these eye conditions that were common were expanded. Some of them included diabetic retinopathy which was reported to affect blood vessels in the light-sensitive tissue called the retina which lines the back of the eye. It was known as the most common cause of vision loss among people with diabetes and the leading cause of vision impairment and blindness among working-age adults. Next up was diabetic macular edema (DME); a consequence of diabetic retinopathy, DME was said to be a swelling in an area of the retina called the macula. Cataract was also discussed. It involved a clouding of the eye's lens. Survey reports suggest that adults with diabetes are two to five times more likely than those without diabetes, to develop cataract. Cataract also tended to develop at an earlier age in people with diabetes. Glaucoma was the next big one. It was described as a group of diseases that damaged the eye's optic nerve—the bundle of nerve fibers that connects the eye to the brain. Some types of glaucoma were associated with elevated pressure inside the eye. In adults, diabetes was reported to nearly double the risk of glaucoma. I found all these at: https://nei.nih.gov/health/diabetic/retinopathy

My eyes were already in a bad state at that point and I did not want to lose my eyesight as my cousin in the Philippines had. I remember her saying it was really difficult living blind. It was as if she was apologizing for not being able to see me after so many years that I finally got to visit her. This shook me badly and I begged her to quit pleading with me over her inability to use her eyes. She died a few years later from complications brought about by diabetes. I truly did not want this because I realized my cousin must have felt she was a big burden to everyone around her. I did not want to be a burden to anyone, especially not to Armie. She had been through a lot already; thanks to my failing health. There was another cousin of mine who passed away after losing his right leg to diabetes. I still remember other friends of mine who lost their legs to diabetes and developed cancer before they died. I did not want to die young. I wanted to live a long and healthy life.

I also looked up the benefits of spinach and I came across medicalnewstoday.com

On this website, Natalie Butler, a corporate dietitian for Apple Inc. in Austin, Texas had reviewed an article about the benefits of spinach and the article said the possible health benefits of consuming spinach included improving blood glucose control in people with diabetes, lowering the risk of cancer, reducing blood pressure, improving bone health, lowering the risk of developing asthma, and more. It asserted that spinach contained an antioxidant known as alpha-lipoic acid which has been proven to lower glucose levels, increase insulin sensitivity, and prevent oxidative stress-induced changes in patients with diabetes, making it a great ally for the management of diabetes. As for cancer management, spinach and other green vegetables was reported to contain chlorophyll which has been shown to be effective at blocking the carcinogenic effects of heterocyclic amines generated when grilling foods at high temperatures. For blood pressure management, spinach's high potassium content was shown to help reduce the effects of sodium in the body. A low potassium intake is just as big of a risk factor for developing high blood pressure as a high sodium intake. I

found   all   these   at
https://www.medicalnewstoday.com/articles/270609.php

I knew bananas and pineapples had their good benefits as well and so taking the TropiKale smoothie every day for the rest of our lives, seemed to be the least gift which Armie and I could give ourselves. Observing this daily routine also improved my self-esteem compared to when I was a meat eater. Then, I never used to pay attention to my health and the impact of the foods I consumed on my general wellbeing. All I cared about then was that the food was delicious, that I was going to be full and satisfied after eating and that I was having fun. With the transition to plant-based diets, I felt responsible and capable of adequately providing myself with the nutritional requirements that my body needed. More importantly was that I was getting a daily regimen of multivitamins without having to bother myself about the dangers of side effects that came with taking multivitamin pills. This is not to say multivitamins pills are bad, but having been manufactured in the laboratory, they must have been stripped off their natural form and anything unnatural cannot be fully absorbed by our body. Even Dr. Raffaella Pernice, my Microbiology professor, recommended that we ate whole vegetables and fruits if we wanted natural vitamins instead of synthetic ones because our body could never fully absorb them. This was during one of our Microbiology classes. There were also speculations of how drugs which were not properly absorbed could escape excretion and go on to form crystals in the kidney, usually referred to as kidney stones.

I looked up the side effects of multivitamins online and stumbled upon NCBI's website. On it, I found their peer-reviewed article, which related that taking high-dose supplements of vitamins A, E, D, C, and folic acid was not always effective for prevention of disease, and that they could even be harmful to the health. NCBI is a credible source because the National Center for Biotechnology Information (NCBI) advances science and health by providing access to biomedical and genomic information.

16

THE JOURNEY CONTINUES

With all the discoveries I had made so far, I still was not satisfied especially with just having the TropiKale smoothie diet and so I continued sourcing new vegan diets online. Luckily, I found many vegan recipes on YouTube. I subscribed to the channels that were committed to developing and introducing vegan diets. I would even do searches on just about any food but would include the keyword 'vegan'. Doing this, I always found someone 'veganizing' almost every recipe I looked up. I also bought a few paperback recipes including "The Prevent and Reverse Heart Disease Cookbook" by Ann and Jane Esselstyn. There were many websites I visited as well and one of my favorite was the forksoverknives.com website. They had hundreds of plant-based vegan recipes. All these searching and finding was a new dimension, which Armie and I found very adventurous as we were constantly trying out new things as far as they were healthy for us. We even decided to spice up our weekends by searching for and exploring vegan restaurants in our area and the recipes they had to offer. We would often compare quality, quantity and innovativeness of the food business owners as we ate in such places, one weekend at a time. We had even reached as far as Philadelphia, Connecticut and New York in search of new vegan diet experiences, and of course, New York City had the most selection of vegan restaurants, in my opinion. You could tell we also enjoyed our lunch dates together. I observed that we started bonding even better and had a lot of endless things to talk about unlike in our previous years of marriage where everyone was too busy trying to make enough bills to support the family and bothering about my then, rapidly declining health.

Although we were having so much fun with this new way of life, I wasn't sure if this whole food plant-based diet would stay with me because everyone I knew had been telling me that eliminating meat from their diet was very difficult and impossible. That was during the first few weeks of transitioning. However, twelve months have gone and I am still vegan. Actually I use the word vegan because many people still do not understand 'Whole Food Plant-Based.' Vegan is the least confusing word to tell people if they ask. Even some people don't know what vegan is. They think it is the same as vegetarian. I don't consider myself to be 100% vegan in the sense that I still use my leather jacket and my favorite Dr. Martens boots which I bought ten years before I decided to switch to a whole food plant-based lifestyle. I heard hardcore vegans never wore anything of animal origin. I'm not that kind of vegan yet but I may not buy anymore leather clothing and apparels.

17

QUICK RESULTS

Three weeks after I stopped eating meat, dairy, fish and eggs, my blood sugar dropped significantly and I was surprised and excited at the same time but I was still skeptical.

"It can't be this quick," I said to myself.

So I continued checking my blood glucose levels twice a day. This was something I used to be scared of doing because of how high my glucose levels used to be when I was still consuming meat-based diets. I continued researching online and watching YouTube video presentations about plant-based diets. Switching to a plant-based lifestyle was not easy, I must confess. It was a struggle for me since I did not start out being a vegan; I grew up eating meat, processed meat, dairy, eggs and fish. I know some people claim that fish is good for us but I stopped eating fish (especially farmed fish such as tilapia and milk fish) because The Physicians Committee for Responsible Medicine asserts that most of the fat in fish is not heart-healthy fat and fish can also be toxic, with dangerous levels of mercury and other pollutants. The commercials and ads were always on television and everywhere I went, including on the subway, the magazines and even on social media. All our friends and families were meat eaters and when we got invited to parties, there were no vegan options. We did not even know what vegan was, back then. After eating plant-based for a month, I began having more energy. I would usually feel rested every morning when I woke up. I used to have a hard time getting up every morning and I would tell Armie to give me fifteen more minutes. That changed after the transition, as my eyes would automatically open at 5:30 am. She even told me that I no longer snored aloud anymore and that I had stopped having nightmares in which I would talk in my sleep. The results of our plant-based diet were showing already.

Another important discovery I learned was Intermittent Fasting (IF) by Dr. Jason Fung, a month after my plant-based diet. Dr. Fung is a Canadian Nephrologist who founded the Intensive Dietary Management Program (IDMP) in Toronto that provides personalized therapeutic nutritional counseling for weight loss and Type 2 Diabetes reversals. He claimed that intermittent fasting was a great way to lose weight quickly.

Intermittent fasting, aka Time Restricted Feeding involved dividing eating and fasting time into two windows; the feeding and fasting windows. According to Dr. Fung, intermittent fasting drops our blood sugar and increases our insulin sensitivity because the digestive system is given a break. So I tried it and my blood sugar level went below a hundred mg/dL every time my body was in a fasted state. Dr. Fung also said that our body burns fat storage for energy while in a fasted state and even more when we exercised. So I started exercising while on fasted state and I kept losing weight. Today, I include intermittent fasting with my vegan lifestyle. Dr. Fung can be found on https://idmprogram.com. This has greatly helped me in promoting my quest for a healthy lifestyle.

18
____

THE VISIT

Three months later, I returned to Dr. Darbouze and told him about my latest discovery. I told him that I had stopped taking my medications because I started eating only plant-based diets and because of this, my blood glucose levels were always normal. I also told him about my newly discovered intermittent fasting. He didn't say anything negative, nor did he try to discourage me. Instead, He told me to monitor my blood sugar everyday and encouraged me to keep doing what I was doing. I did my blood work that day and my Hemoglobin A1c was 7.1. It was 9.9 three months before I started the plant-based diet. So the plant-based diet had helped drop my HbA1c by 2.8 points in three months and this got me really motivated. I also lost 35 pounds, although most of it was probably water. I was very happy with the results and continued eating plant-based diet and continued exercising regularly. Today, I'm 165 pounds and my Hemoglobin A1c is 5.5, which is normal. My LDL cholesterol and triglycerides levels are also normal. And now, I've been eating plant-based diets for about a year now, I don't take any medication, and I'm still going to lose weight and feel great.

19

———

CONFESSIONS

Did I have any struggles in the beginning while making the transition?

Yes it was a very huge struggle because I grew up eating all these unhealthy delicious foods. Our dishes were heavily meat-based and the fact that I became obsessed about them, owing largely to how I did not get enough meat in my meals during my childhood, also made it difficult to so easily switch to whole food plant-based diets. Meat and meat products were and are always on television as well as everywhere I went. All our friends and families were meat eaters and when we got invited to parties, there were no vegan options. Another very strong factor was that I did not know what to eat when I transitioned but through dogged determination and sheer inquisitiveness, I was able to achieve good success with my new food lifestyle.

How long did it take before I started noticing results?

I started noticing results within three weeks!

What were the first results I noticed?

I observed that my blood sugar level decreased significantly, my energy levels increased greatly and that I lost some weight.

Has making this transition changed my life for the better?

A very big yes! My life is definitely better as I no longer have fears of dying young or too early. I am more positive about life and even more excited to take on new projects seeing as I have the chance to live longer as well as that I am usually more energized than I used to be while I was still a meat eater. I do not have to live on pills and insulin injections and that is so amazing because I would no longer have bruises. I even save more now that I am not buying medications worth hundreds of dollars of medicine. I am definitely living a healthier lifestyle; looking and feeling better each day.

What is my life right now?

I'm still in the learning process; still reading and researching about nutrition because I'm not out of the woods yet. I still have twenty pounds to lose to achieve my ideal weight of 145. I am also going to attempt long fasting. In fact, I am currently on day one of my five-day water fast and my wife is with me on this, but generally, my life is way better than it was before I watched the "What the Health" documentary. I am really excited about my life right now.

What would my three biggest tips for readers considering taking on this lifestyle, be?

Tip 1: Read, research and learn all you can about the whole food plant-based lifestyle. YouTube has very helpful videos by Dr. Michael Greger, Dr. Klaper, Dr. Neal Barnard, Dr. John McDougall, Dr. Caldwell Esselstyn, and Dr. T. Collin Campbell. These doctors will tell you everything you need to know. Information is key to living a long healthy life, in fact it is necessary to all parts of life. With information you can change the world, at least your world.

Tip 2: Identify your purpose and the things that motivate you. I think it is easier to succeed in anything if you have a purpose and motivation that drives you. This way, you can be willing to give up some habits because you surely know what you would like to achieve with this new food lifestyle. If you don't have something motivating you to push through, you will soon fall off the wagon.

Tip 3: Properly document your own transformation. Your failures and successes; every single step you take, document them for future references. Join plant-based community groups on social media so that you can be inspired by other people's growth. This would help you appreciate your progress while sharing it with support groups that has the same interest as you. Plant Fit Movement on Facebook is my favorite group created by Luke Tan, a plant-based proponent who is supportive and inspiring. Also, you may likely find encouragement from other people's success stories and this may be a great motivation tool for your own journey towards a healthier lifestyle.

20

WHAT THEY WOULD NEVER TELL YOU ABOUT DIABETES

The pharmaceutical and medical industry has for years been in the business of taking care of patients and managing health challenges and conditions. We have glorified our doctors and other medical practitioners for the great job they have been doing in saving human lives and the entire human race, if we should judge from the big picture.

However, there is more beyond the big picture. Within it lie hidden truths most doctors would never tell you. Medical bodies and certain organizations would never tell you that something as basic as the food you eat can greatly influence your health as much as curing your ailments. They would never tell you this because the aim is to keep you coming again and again for medications and consultation, which are often very expensive especially if you do not have access to free or highly subsidized medical services.

What they would never tell you about diabetes is that Type 2 Diabetes is absolutely reversible. The myth that you were bound to live with diabetes once you had it till you kicked the bucket, is one of the greatest lies of the past few centuries.

Withholding such information from the masses is essential in keeping medical practitioners in business and nobody wants to be out of business. It is such a sad thing but more importantly, you now know what they never wished that you knew.

Even most fast food business owners are aware that their meat-based cuisines had a major role to play in the development of diabetes, but even they have to stay in business or face burning out. This is why such industries pump in lots of funds into marketing their brands and products, annually. Everywhere you go, you are bound to get flooded with images of one. They know that the mind is easily stimulated and influenced by what it sees, especially if the act is repeated consistently over time.

Pharmaceutical industries are not left out. Ever wondered why they still put a lot of resources into advertising their drugs to you? It is because they know that medicine is a very serious business which has over time being able to convince all of us that we need something extra, drugs, if we must maintain good health. And as long as they can uphold this, they were sure to never fizzle out of business.

Healthy living goes beyond having buckets of ice cream and lots of meat and meat products in your diets. Barbecues are a lovely way of hanging out with family and friends. However, such practice when observed on a regular basis can cause outcomes more damaging than all the fun and satisfaction you could ever get from eating grilled meat.

There is a lot you stand to gain when you embrace a whole food plant-based diets lifestyle. The benefits range from healthier organ functioning to anti-aging and most importantly, you would have a low risk tendency of having a metabolic disease. What could be more beautiful than living life to the fullest knowing that you did not have to live, swallowing large numbers of pills that had their very own side effects, every day of your life?

What you eat can heal or kill you. You have to decide which way it would go. You are solely responsible for your health; you are responsible for living a long, fulfilling life. The question is are you taking responsibility of your health?

Compare these!

Having all the pork, beef, chicken, eggs, cheese, yogurt and others, and then going on to have diabetes, which you would have to manage with drugs till the last day you saw the sun rise.

And...

Eating only plant-based diets, constantly feeling rejuvenated and more without having to live on pills that would take up a large part of your budget.

Which would you prefer?

I think I know which of the two options above your mind is going for. The only challenge would lie in switching from just any kind of diet to a more conscious whole food plant-based lifestyle. And while I will not say that it is so easy especially if you are a meat lover like I was, I can assure you that it is possible and not impossible as some friends told me. As you have seen from my story in which I have narrated my journey from the time when I was healthy, down to my struggle with weight loss and diabetes and finally, at my healthy plant-based lifestyle, negligence was a major problem that deterred my health's improvement. And even though the pills were never going to be a better option than a total switch to whole-food plant-based diets, I could have still saved myself the stress if I had exercised more and ate more healthily.

The first hurdle facing you is making up your mind about whether you truly want to take back the charge you once had of your health and life. Once you do that, everything you do and every step you take would be geared at ensuring that you are constantly seeking new ways to live healthy. You may worry about the limited food options before you but like I have said YouTube holds a lot of video presentations featuring do it yourself sessions of people 'veganizing' almost any meal you look up.

This is also an opportunity for you to be more creative about your food recipes. There are endless things to do with vegetables, salads.

EPILOGUE

I am very happy that you have made it to this point and I commend your persistence. It goes to show that you have all the strength to make those lifestyle changes that you need to take charge of your life. Changes like eating the right kind of diets you have learnt is best for the human system, in this book. You now know about my journey towards a healthy lifestyle from which I truly hope that you have learnt.

Avoid eating meat, processed meat, dairy, eggs and fish. Avoid simple sugars such as sodas, juices and candies. Stop smoking and drinking alcohol. Include a weekly exercise in your schedule by walking at least thirty minutes daily or join the gym. If you are not pregnant, intermittent fasting will help you lose weight and become insulin sensitive. Eating two meals a day is better compared to eating three meals a day because it gives our digestive system a break; but if you must eat three meals a day, avoid eating snacks in between meals because eating this will raise your insulin levels every time. If you are taking diabetic medication, tell your doctor about intermittent fasting so he can adjust your medication. Taking Metformin while doing intermittent fasting may cause your blood sugar level to drop really low and cause Hypoglycemia. I stopped taking Metformin without my doctor's consent because of this. I learned that some hormones in our body such as glucagon would keep our blood sugar level in homeostasis. Adopt a whole food plant-based lifestyle.

I believe that Type 2 Diabetes and obesity are not hereditary. It is following our parents' bad food choices that cause the disease. I believe it is the lack of education, proper dissemination of information, understanding and the accumulation of our bad habits that have resulted in our metabolic diseases. We may come from different backgrounds and culture, speak different languages, have different looks. But we all have a common anatomy and physiology, and we also have the same choices when it comes to our health.

Diabetes and obesity does not discriminate; it doesn't care about our culture or background or age. It only respects and gives way to people who have determined in their hearts to embrace healthier eating lifestyles.

I know you are one of these people and that this may mark the beginning of a turnaround in your health. Therefore, I congratulate you in advance for the giant strides you will achieve by putting to use, all that you have learnt from this book. If I could defeat Type 2 diabetes and turn my life around for the better despite the odds, I bet you can too. The secret is in your food.

www.ingramcontent.com/pod-product-compliance
Lightning Source LLC
Chambersburg PA
CBHW070043260726
48658CB00002B/701